Table of contents

Garrow – Millet

Garrow is a type of grain that grows in mainland Somaliland, and it is often consumed during breakfast or for dinner. In the West, it is comparable to the coarser grain of the couscous, and it is available in Somali food markets. Garrow, also called millet, can be eaten in different ways. You can eat the Garrow as it comes, in coarser form, but you can also throw it in the food processor and mix it to a finer grain. It turns into a porridge, or it converts into a pancake. The amount of nutrients and vitamins in this type of grain is underestimated. Garrow is filled with fibres, calcium, and antioxidants, which gives you an energy boost and does not contain gluten.

Furthermore, this type of grain contains minerals like iron, potassium, and several vitamin B's. In the West, this would be comparable to the gluten-free breakfast wheat that is to be found in the cereal aisle of the supermarket. Because of the warm climate in Somaliland, it's common to eat a quick warm meal in the morning, an elaborate warm meal in the afternoon, and a light meal for dinner.

Necessities: for three people
-500 gram Millet
-Water
-Somali butter
(Available in Somali stores)
-Milk
-Sugar

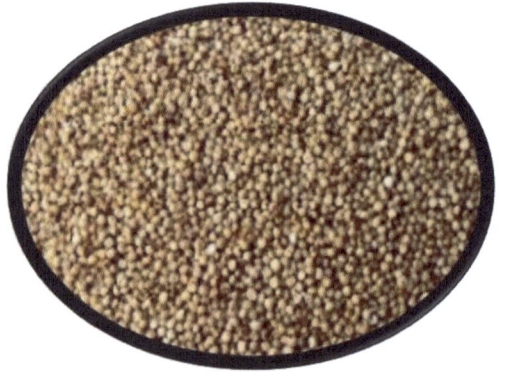

Millet Seed

Preparation:
Boil approximately 500 grams of millet in a saucepan with water. Stir while the millet is cooking in the water on low fire. Turn off the heat after 5 minutes and place the lid on the pan to let the millet simmer for a bit. According to personal preference and taste, you can add a teaspoon of butter, a little bit of sugar, and milk to the Garrow. The Garrow can also be eaten with yoghurt

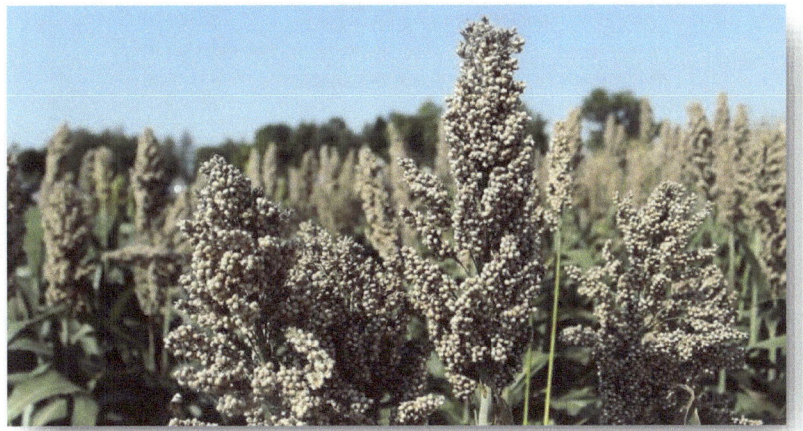

Millet plant

and dates, which on their own also contain high nutritional values. It is also delicious to eat it with sliced banana and chia seeds.

Delightful Somali recipes

Garrow with blueberries and Chia Seeds

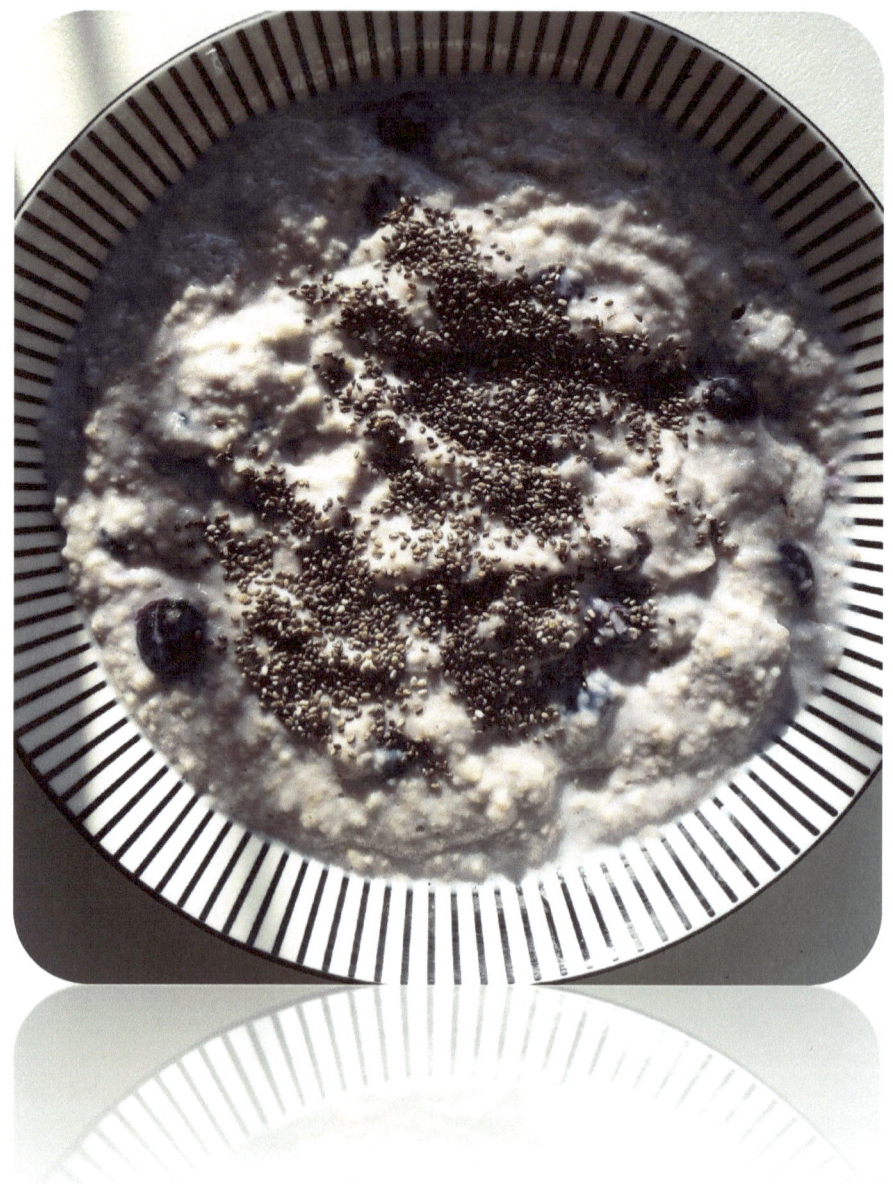

Delightful Somali recipes

Kaljo - Kidney dish

It is normal to eat organ meats such as liver, heart, kidney for breakfast in Somaliland. What makes eating entrails so unique, except, of course, for its health benefits, is that it's eaten for breakfast. For Somalis, a good breakfast is essential because for them, especially those that are not living in the West, the morning is the longest part of the day. For example, their workday starts at 7 am and ends approximately at 1 pm. People head home to have an elaborate cooked lunch consisting of meat, rice or pasta then take a siesta to avoid being in the sun when it's at its highest or working in an area with no air-conditioning then go back to work from 3 pm onwards till 7 pm in most cases. It is a habit to purchase fresh organic meat and biological offal meats like Kaljo and kidneys every morning within the Somali culture. Since most people are dependent on generators for electricity, it's uncommon to refrigerate the meat for more extended periods. Besides that, the Somali is very particular about their meat and even conceited as they believe in the idea of refrigerated meat being lousy meat. The Somali wholeheartedly believes that the nutrients in the meat get lost once it has been refrigerated, especially when the meat has been stored for longer than one day. So fresh produce and organic (bio-meats) poultry, meat, and fish have precedence amongst the population. In particular, the kidneys (Kaljo) of a camel, goat, or sheep are popular due to their filling component, nutritional value, and quick and easy preparation manner.

Compared to the Western culture in the Somali culture, eating organ meat is an ordinary course of business because people have easier access to these meats.
Kaljo, which translates to kidneys in English, contains many essential nutrients and proteins, such as niacin, copper, magnesium, zinc, iron, and vitamins B-3, 6,12, A, D.

Delightful Somali recipes

Moreover, here in the West, meat often contains hormones, which directly affect the animal's organs. So amongst the Somalis in the West, eating offal is unpopular. Unless one lives on a farm, owns cattle, and has access to organic meat, the general advice is to not consume organ meat.

Necessities:
- 500 grams of fresh Kaljo (kidney) can consist of a calf/goat/camel (organic)
- 1 to 2 Onion
- 1 Tomato
- 2 gloves of garlic
- 1 red chili (Piri Piri/Carolina cayenne)
- 1 or 2 Green pepper (banana pepper)
- coriander (optional)
- 1 teaspoon salt
- 1 teaspoon Black pepper
- 150 ml Sunflower oil/butter/ Somali butter (made from sheep FAT) Somali butter is available in Somali grocery shops.
* Casserole/frying pan

Preparation:
Take a frying pan, heat one tablespoon of Somali butter, or if you are in the West, 100 grams of dairy butter or 150 ml sunflower oil should be sufficient. Leave the butter or oil to melt in the pan and let it swelter. Add the diced onion, two gloves of garlic, one sliced tomato, a finely chopped couple of green banana peppers, and the red chilli pepper. Depending on your taste, either one of the peppers, green or red, can be hot. Generally speaking, the red cayenne or Piri Piri peppers are hotter in taste than their green counterparts. The spice gives the entrails meat that little bit of extra flavour. Although the Kaljo (kidney) is somewhat challenging to chew on than the Beerr (liver), it is crucial to not bake the kidneys for too long. A couple of minutes are just enough to preserve all the nutrients. Therefore, it's essential to add the Kaljo together with the vegetables quickly; this way, you

Delightful Somali recipes

will allow all the juices to come together to melt beautifully together.

Bake this for 3 minutes, and it's done.

You can sprinkle some finely chopped fresh coriander and green pepper over it for an aesthetic presentation, that is when you are ready to serve your dish. If you don't like coriander, parsley, or just the green pepper will suffice. With this, it is essential not to take the hot peppers because that would be the first thing you will get into your mouth, and that will overwhelm your taste buds and ruin the taste of the entire dish.

Beerr – Liver dish

Liver or Beerr in the Somali language is a precarious piece of meat consumed for breakfast in Somaliland. Because Somaliland is an Islamic country, the day starts relatively early. Most people get up early for the Morning Prayer; after the prayer, most fresh food store owners open their stores. And so you can do all groceries for the rest of the day, provided that you had already decided what you want to eat for that day. In case you weren't able to make up your mind, there is nothing to worry about as you can at least buy fresh sheep, camel, or goat liver at the butcher for your breakfast.

The liver is a delicate piece of meat that is at its best when consumed fresh, so without it being refrigerated for too long. Even a day in the refrigerator makes the liver lose nutrients and its natural taste. The Somalis do not like to consume meat that has been refrigerated for even one day. They want their meat fresh. Just like other organ meats, the liver is a fine entrails meat that's light enough to eat for breakfast. Yet it's packed with minerals such as iron, zinc, selenium, copper, niacin, and vitamins such as A, B-6 & B-12, B-3, and (D) that you will need to get healthy through the day. So it is not a bad idea to have the liver for breakfast. In addition, you do get a full feeling which will easily last you for the rest of the day.

In general, under the Somali people in the West, eating offal is not very popular because it's pretty tricky to get fresh meat or meat that does not contain hormones.

Necessities:
- 500 grams of fresh Beerr (liver)
- 2 Onion (white/Red)
- 1 Tomato
- 1 green chili pepper (Serrano)

Delightful Somali recipes

- 1 Red chilli powder (mild)
- fresh coriander
- ½ teaspoon Salt
- 1 teaspoon Black pepper
- Somali butter/50 ml sunflower oil/50 grams butter
* Casserole

Preparation:
Cut two white or red onions into small blocks, cut the 500 grams of the liver into pieces, do the same with the 2-green peppers and the fresh tomato.

In addition, you put 50 grams butter, 1 tsp red chilli powder, salt, and pepper within easy reach because you are going to need that too.

Heat one tablespoon melted butter or 50 grams butter or sunflower oil in a casserole. Then add the pre-cut onions, let the onions bake for a minute, then add the diced tomato and green pepper. Because of their heat component, hot green chilli peppers smell spicy, and if you inhale that hot-pepper aroma, unlike with the onions, you don't cry, but you will cough due to the gasses coming off the peppers.

Slowly start stirring this mixture, add the coriander and shortly after, add the liver to the mix and keep stirring it. Lastly, add a pinch of salt and let it all come together for about a minute and a half, two minutes, and voilà you just got yourself the healthiest breakfast possible.

For an aesthetic whole, you can now choose to cut one or two fresh red peppers, not hot ones, but for example, a Banana pepper or an Anaheim, and scatter that over the dish. Or if you don't like spicy food, or you want people to enjoy this dish that cannot handle spicy food, choose not to bake the chilli pepper in the container, rather chop that very fine and sprinkle it to your taste over the dish. Scattering a few coriander leaves over this dish always makes up for a beautiful picture.

Delightful Somali recipes

Wadneh – Heart Dish

For many people, the idea of consuming offal meat and especially the heart of an animal, sounds disgusting. However, this is just in our heads because eating organ meat has many health benefits, and it is also lean and clean, therefore safe for consumption. The heart of a sheep, goat, cow, or camel is an organ with a unique taste that your taste butts need some time to adjust to. Once it is prepared well and regularly included in your diet, you will enjoy the tremendous health benefits this organ carries within itself. For example, it contains protein, minerals, and vitamins such as vitamin B2, B6, B12, selenium, iron, phosphorus, zinc, thiamine, folate, and magnesium.

When buying entrails meat in general, it's best to buy the heart, liver, or kidney from organic, i.e., biological or grass-fed animals who had a free-range life.

Requirements: 3/4 people
- 500 grams of the grass-fed animal heart (depending on one own preference, this could be the heart from a calf/cow, sheep, goat, or even a camel)
- 1 or 2 Onions (red or white does not matter)
- 2 Tomato
- 2 gloves of garlic
- 1 Red/green (hot) chilli pepper (cayenne)
- green pepper, not hot (Anaheim)
- 1 bell pepper (colour does not matter)
- parsley
- Salt
- Black pepper
- Sunflower oil/butter / Somali butter made from cow/sheep fat
* casserole or frying pan

Preparation:
Pre-heat a bit of butter in a casserole or a deep frying pan—mix two gloves of garlic with some cumin seeds in a blender or mortar. Add sliced vegetables such as onions, tomatoes, red chilli peppers, and cumin and garlic paste. Let this bake for a minute, then add the diced wander, the heart to the mixture. Stir the mixture so the aromas can evenly spread juices throughout the entire dish. Lastly, add a little bit of pepper and salt to the mix, and your breakfast is ready within two to three minutes. For aesthetics, sprinkle some parsley leaves over the meat.
In Somaliland, this dish is often served and eaten with un-sweetened thin pancakes or savoury Sabayad, Somali flatbread.

Loxoox – Pancakes

The most popular breakfast in Somaliland is Loxoox, pronunciation logoog, or thin pancakes made from yeast, flour, and water or milk and baked in a flat heavy-metal pancake pan with no sides, called Dawwa. The Loxoox mix does not contain eggs per se. It is common in Somaliland for families to pre-mix the flour and water in a bowl in the evening and let it rise overnight. Due to the overall warm and mellow weather, the flour mix increases well.

requisites: 4 people
- 250 grams of plain flour
- 4 eggs (optional)
- 200 ml of water
- Salt - Sugar
- Somali butter (from the Somali store)
- Sunflower oil
* Dawwa
* Cloth

Preparation:
As stated above, mix flour with water and yeast and let it sit for a while. In the West, you can buy the pre-mixed pancake mixes or add eggs, milk, or water to it and use a blender or a hand mixture to mix it all.
Somalilanders beat the dough with their hand, or they let the blender do the job for them. And it's not common to add eggs to the flower, but it's optional. The mixture usually exists of flour, yeast, and water.
When the cooking process starts, you scoop out the fluid mixture with a cup and then make circles with the bottom of that cup to spread the mixture evenly throughout the Dawwa until you get a perfect 360-degree ring. The consistency is thicker in the middle and thins out towards the outside of the circle. But it is not that

Delightful Somali recipes

thick, at least not to the extent where the dough in the middle is still raw. It thins out on the outside, but the mixture is evenly spread, so circles come to existence, dividing the processes that look like little traffic bumps but then soft and squishy. Throughout the pancake, there will be air bubbles in the mixture. Therefore you don't need to turn around the pancake and bake it on both sides. Baking it on one side is enough.

The great thing about this pancake is that it can be eaten with a savoury sauce made from offal meat like kidney or liver, but it will taste good with just a little bit of sugar and butter drizzled over it. The latter is popular amongst children as they haven't developed a taste for spicy food yet, so sprinkling a bit of sugar and drizzling melted butter over their pancakes is tasty enough for them.

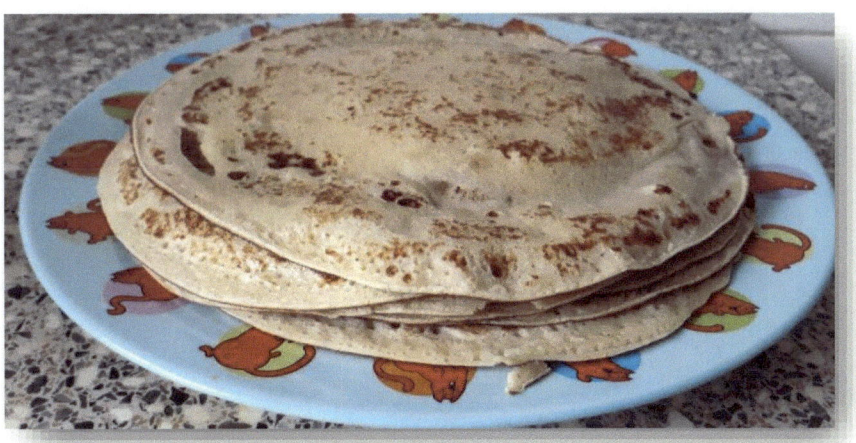

Loxoox

Delightful Somali recipes

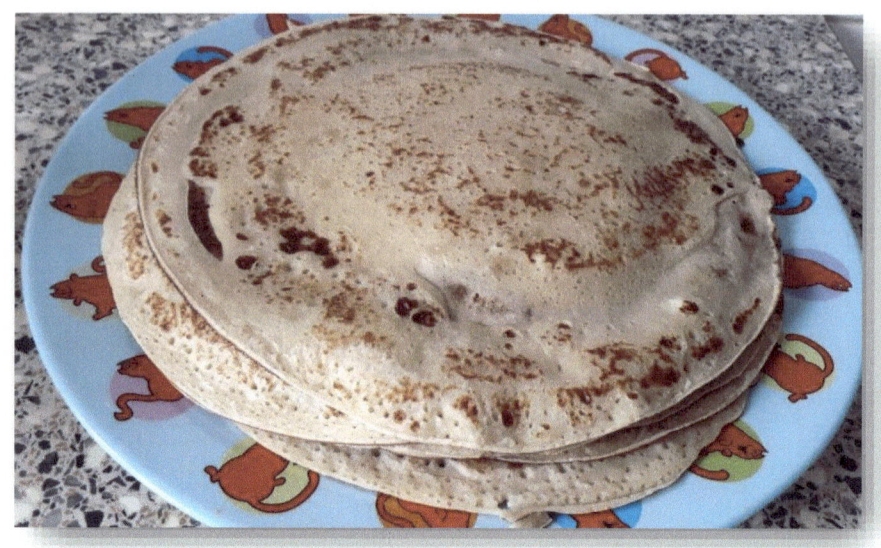

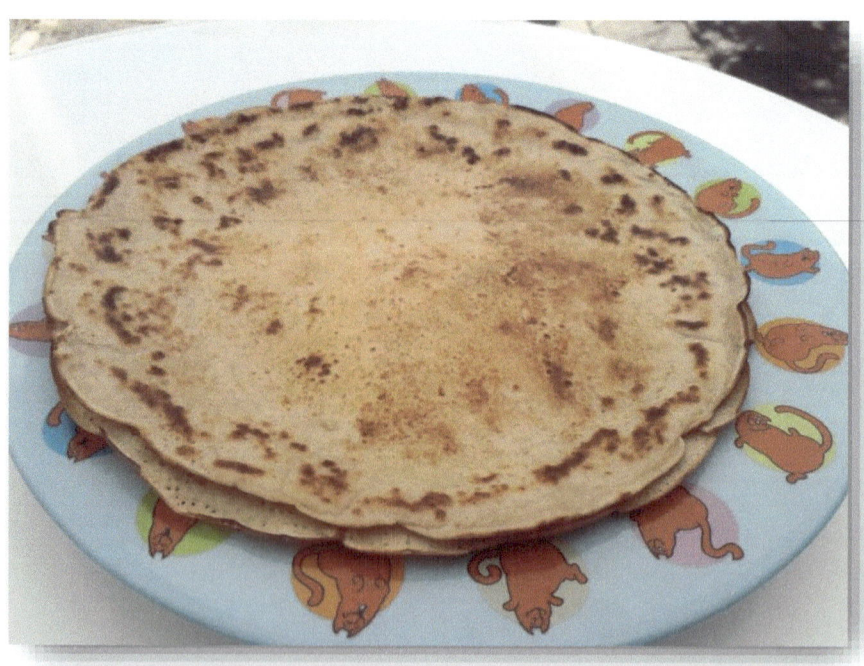

Delightful Somali recipes

Roodi iyo baíd (pan-fried toast) – Eggs & bread

Roodi is the Somali word for bread. We are talking about bread with eggs or eggs with bread as the two in this dish are intertwined. It is pretty standard for families in Somaliland to have goats or chickens, a few sheep, or even camels if you own a large piece of land. Most families have goats and chickens for milk, meat, eggs, and even business purposes; this is mainly the case with nomadic families. However, city people also keep chickens or a goat or two but not for business; instead, it is just for personal consumption. Eggs are included in the breakfast or dinner of the Somali diet. Having eggs for dinner might sound odd to many people, but dinner is a small meal in Somaliland. People tend to eat a warm and elaborate lunch and something practical, often easy for dinner.

Necessities: 2 people
- 4 eggs
- 4 to 5 slices of bread / smaller pieces in case of a baguette
- ½ cup Milk
- ½ teaspoon Salt
- ½ teaspoon of black pepper
- 200 grams Butter / 150 ml sunflower oil
*Bowl
*fry pan

Preparation:
Grab a bowl and use a tablespoon or a whisker to whisk the eggs; while whisking the eggs, add salt and pepper to the mixture. Add about 125 ml of milk to the eggs and whisk a couple more minutes until the colour of the substance changes into a beautiful yellow colour. Then dip the bread in the mixture of eggs and milk. Leave the bread in there for 2 seconds so the bread can absorb the milk, turn it around, so the bread gets the chance to soak in the milk on both sides.

Delightful Somali recipes

Put some butter or sunflower oil in a pan and heat it well. Dip the bread in the oil and fry it on both sides, approximately a minute per side. If you leave the bread slightly longer than a minute in the oil, it might burn because the outer layer consists of eggs and milk burns quicker than the bread. Moreover, the oil is also heating up as you are frying the bread.

If you are making this dish for small children, they might appreciate a sweeter version of this pan-fried toast, so adding sugar or using condensed milk might do the job but leave the black pepper out in that case.

Sabayad – Flat Bread

Sabayad is a savoury pastry dish similar to a double-sided roti from the Indian, Pakistani kitchen. This is a versatile product that can be eaten in many different ways. The most simplistic way to eat this dish is with butter and honey or sugar to replace the honey. It's common to serve this dish that way to children for breakfast, lunch, or even dinner. In contrast, adults prefer to eat this dish with a spicy sauce, often made of minced meat and some vegetables or with suqaar.

Requirements:
- dough rolling pin
- plastic foil
- 0.5 gram Yeast
- 500 grams plain delicate flour (let it go through a sieve)
- 250 ml sunflower oil
- 1 cup of water (250ml)
- ½ teaspoon salt

Preparation:
Put 500 grams of refined flour and yeast together with a little bit of water, approximately 1/3 of a cup (83ml), in a bowl. Immediately add half a teaspoon of salt and start kneading it. You can add a tablespoon of sunflower oil to prevent the dough from sticking to your hand and the bowl as you knead.
Continue kneading until a compact, coherent soft roll of dough comes about. It should now be safe to stick your fingers or thumb into this dough roll, and it will not stick to your hands. Instead, you're able to see a handprint on the dough and even form shapes with it. Leave the dough roll to rest for a while (an hour or two).

Divide the dough into smaller pieces with your hands and roll it between the palms off your hands to form round mushy parts, like a meatball but then from the dough. Sprinkle some flour on the counter to prevent your dough balls from sticking to the kitchen work-top. Cover it with plastic foil.

Grab a rolling pin, sprinkle some flour on the work surface, and roll out the dough balls one by one. Occasionally take some plain flour between the tips of your fingers and sprinkle it on your workbench and top of the flat surface of the rolled-out flour. This is especially good to prevent the dough from sticking to your rolling pin or kitchen counter/ workbench. If done correctly, the dough is moist enough but not wet, so it will not stick to your hands easily or leave a gluey substance to anything you're working with.
While rolling out the dough, make sure you turn it a couple of times, roll out the sides, and allow your sabayad to be evenly flattened out on every side. If all goes well, you will get a brilliant rectangular flatbread evenly thin on all sides.

Place a flat pan, like a pancake pan – Dawwa in Somali but heavier from your regular pancake pan with no sides, on high heat. Grease the pan with a bit of Somali butter or regular butter; if you are in the West, melt the butter and make sure the butter is not thick but richly smeared over the pan. The tip of a teaspoon will do. Wipe the butter off a little bit to avoid oil getting absorbed by the dough, causing oily patches on the Sabayad. If this happens and the rest of your flatbread is not fried yet, you might even get burned patches of dough on your flatbread. Then place the rolled dough on the Dawwa but stay close to it so you can press down the sides with a spatula or with your hand holding a small cloth. This allows the bread to be baked evenly on all sides. When one side is baked nice and brown, turn the bread around.

The people of Somaliland have the option to cook and bake on gas or charcoal; the latter mainly happens in the countryside amongst nomads. The exciting thing about cooking on charcoal is that your food, in this case, the Sabayad, does get a grill-like barbeque-esk flavour without it being overwhelming. And

Delightful Somali recipes

because the flames you are cooking on are more robust, your food cooks in a shorter time frame. While cooking on gas, many smoke comes out of the kitchen, but the taste is very different. The Sabayad cooked on gas tastes less robust than the one cooked on charcoal.

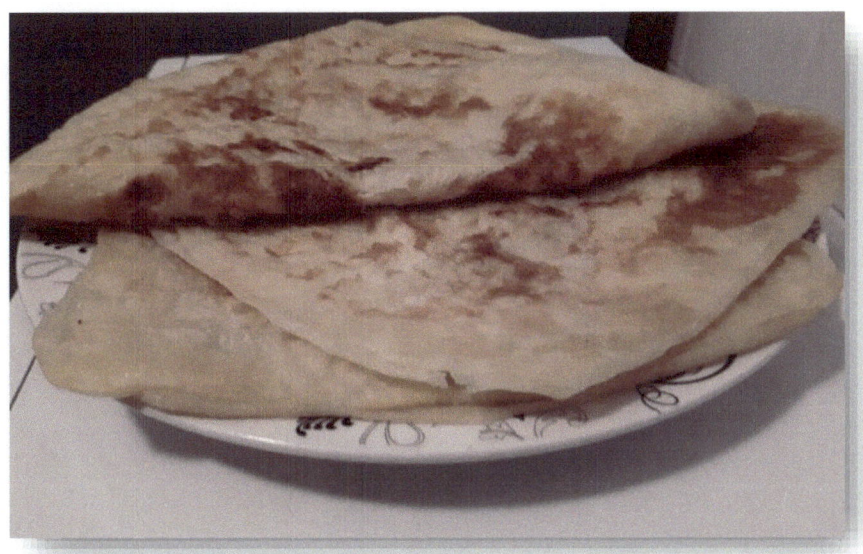

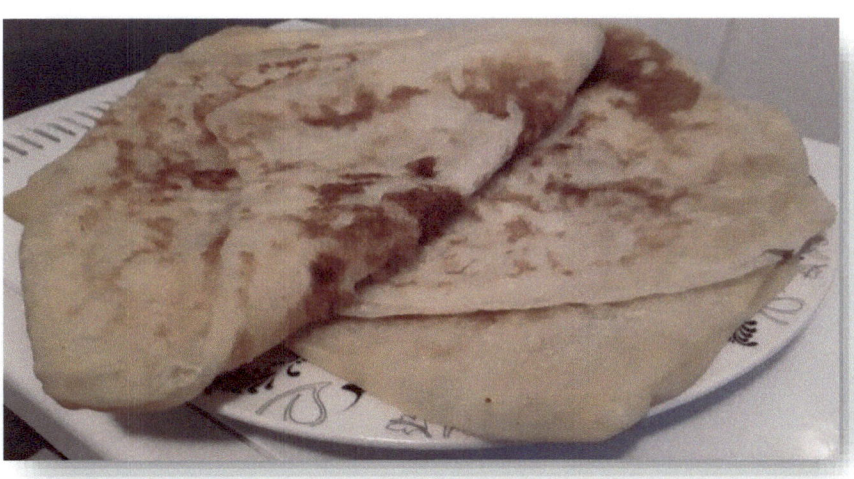

Sabayad

Delightful Somali recipes

Suqaar – Beef Stew

Somalis are meat eaters and can eat meat for breakfast, lunch, and dinner. This is one of these Somali meat dishes that are easy to make yet very versatile as it's easy to combine with different dishes in the form of a side dish or as gravy. On top of that, it is delicious and nourishing.

requisites: 3 people
- 500 grams of lean beef
- 1 red onion
- 1 large or two small tomatoes (peeled)
- 150 ml sunflower oil
- 50 ml butter
- 1 teaspoon of black pepper
- 1 teaspoon of salt
- black cumin seeds
- 1 red bell pepper
- 1 green chilli pepper (Jalapeno)
- 2 garlic gloves
- little bit of coriander leaves
* wok pan

Preparation:
Put two peeled garlic gloves in a mortar along with a ½ teaspoon of cumin seeds and a little bit of coriander. Grind this into a paste-like substance and put it apart as you will need it a little bit later.
Slice the beef into medium-sized cubes and put that on the stove in a wok pan together with 250 ml of water on medium heat. Cook the pieces of meat for approximately 10 minutes until it excretes all its moisture and the water evaporates. Poor 50 ml of sunflower oil over the meat cubes and fry it for 5 minutes on its own. Then add the garlic, cumin, and coriander paste and add the cube size onions and 50 ml of melted butter. After a minute, add

a teaspoon of black pepper, chopped serrano, and a teaspoon of salt. Cook the tomatoes in water until the skin starts to come off, remove it from the stove, and peel the tomatoes. The tomatoes should still be hard enough to slice and not yet at the status of mushy. Slice the bell pepper into small cubes and add both the tomatoes and the bell peppers to the mixture of meat and spices. Add about 200 ml of water to the beef and leave it for another 7 minutes.

This easy-to-make dish can be enjoyed with roodi (Somali bread), Sabayad (Somali flatbread), or with Loxoox (Somali pancakes), provided you crave this in the morning for breakfast. It also goes well with white rice and pasta, although in that case, the suqaar should contain slightly more moisture.

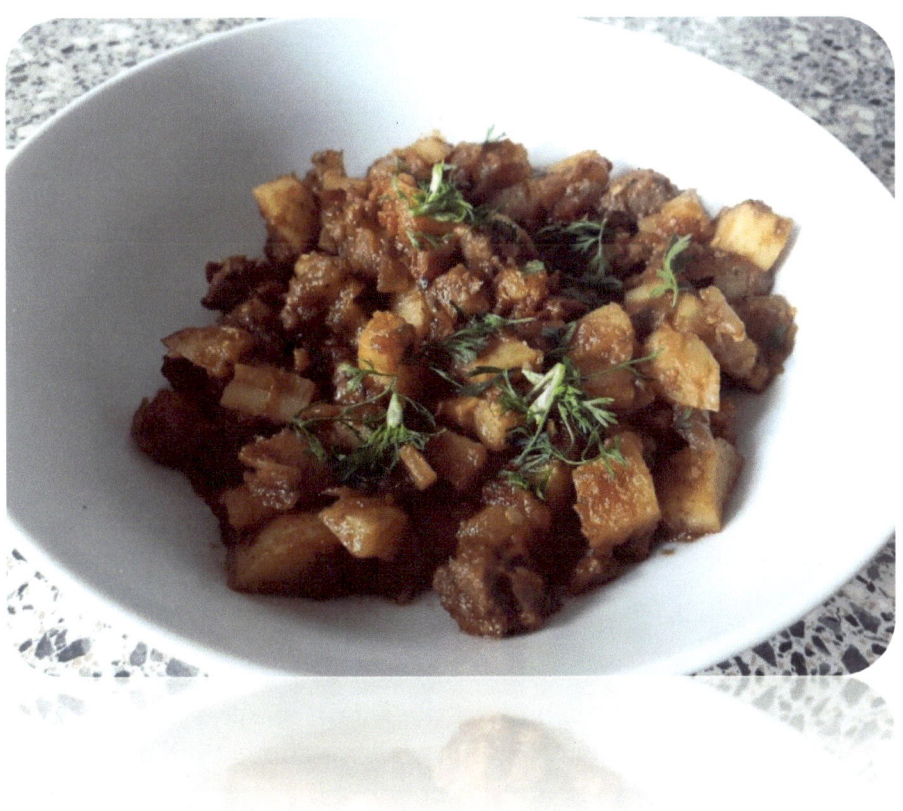

Suqaar with Barado
Delightful Somali recipes

Barad'o Iyo Kaluun – Potato & Salmon

Somali potato dish with salmon is a convenient dish with a healthy amount of minerals and other nutritional values. It is filling and usually eaten by Somalis to add variety to their diet and often on their rest-from-eating-meat day.

Necessities: 3 people
- approximately seven large floury potatoes
- 3 pieces of wild salmon
- 3 white onions
- 50 g butter
- 3 Red chillies (Serrano)
- 2 tablespoons of sunflower oil
- ½ teaspoon of salt
- teaspoon of Curry powder

Preparation:
Put three pieces of red peppers in a blender or mortar. Use the pestle to mash the chilli into a paste-like substance.
Cut the onions into cubes, peel the potatoes, and cut them into coarse (oval) pieces. Poor tiny bit of water in a frying pan and some of the chilli pepper paste, lay the three slices of salmon fillet in the frying pan. Let the salmon cook on low fire for about 10 minutes, turn it halfway around to evenly cook the salmon on the sides. To prevent the salmon from sticking to the pan, add a little bit of sunflower oil to the pan and add pepper and salt. There is no need to put a lid on the frying pan.

Put the potatoes and onions together with 1 litre of water in a saucepan. Add a little bit of curry, a dash of salt, and 50g butter. Put the lid on the pan and let it cook for about 15 minutes. Occasionally stir the potatoes but do this gently as you don't want to break the potatoes.

As the curry and the onions melt together, delicious aromas are released, creating a smooth set of soft gravy for the potatoes. The potatoes are not pureed but have kept their form and are soft.

* Tip: This dish can also be made without curry powder.

Duqad Iyo baíd – Spiced minced with egg

The Somali is very resourceful in terms of their food combinations. One thing that they dread leaving out of their breakfast or lunch in Somaliland is meat. This particular dish is made out of fried beef, minced beef or goat minced, and eggs and is often eaten for breakfast or lunch in Somaliland. Somalilanders residing in the West with busy schedules tend to make this dish on the weekends for lunch or dinner after their nine to five jobs.

This seemingly odd combination of minced eggs and spices is dense with essential vitamins and minerals. Beef minced contains a good amount of vitamin B3, B6, B12, selenium, zinc, phosphorus, and iron.
Goat meat is slightly healthier than beef meat as it contains fewer calories due to its lean nature, resulting in less saturated fats and higher nutritional value. For example, there is more iron in goat meat than there is in beef meat. Goat meat also contains vitamin B6, B12, vitamin C, D, and A and calcium, magnesium, and potassium.
Goat meat has a lower cholesterol level than other red meat and can perfectly be combined with eggs. If one is suffering from heart disease or high cholesterol, goat meat is a safer choice than other red meat.
According to the food and health guidelines, one large egg accounts for 2/3 of adults' daily recommended cholesterol intake.

Eggs form a great source of protein, but they also contain healthy fats and tremendous amounts of vitamin B. B2, B5, B6, B12. A good portion of vitamin C, vitamin D, vitamin E, vitamin K. Moreover eggs also contain minerals like zinc, folate, phosphorus, and selenium. The health components in eggs are often underrated and crossed over by their high cholesterol content. However, eggs help fight diseases like muscle degeneration and even increase memory due to their choline content.

Overall this dish is packed with necessary protein and recently discovered nutrients like choline in eggs, so go ahead and include them into your diet.

Necessities: 2 people
- 4 eggs
- 200 grams off goat minced/beef minced
- 1 large regular union
- ½ teaspoon Salt
- ½ teaspoon of cumin powder
- ½ teaspoon red chilli powder
- ½ teaspoon of mixed black and white pepper
- ½ teaspoon coriander powder
- 4 gloves of garlic
- 150 grams Butter / 100 ml sunflower oil
*fry pan

Preparation:
Preheat approximately 100 ml of sunflower oil or 150 grams of butter; mind you, the minced will release its natural fats, so you just need a little bit of oil or butter for this dish. Place the 200 grams of preferred minced meat in the pan and let it simmer for a good five minutes. If you are using minced that is not fresh, detangle the small lumps with a spoon while on the stove. Add the garlic and a pinch of salt to the minced.

Cut the onion into small cubes and add that to the minced in the pan. Once the onions start to change, colour, add the powdered spices and stir it well. Also, add a little bit of water to your minced spice mixture, that will allow the minced meat to absorb more off the spices and let it simmer until the little bit of water disappears from your pan.

While this is happening, crack four eggs in a bowl, add a hinge of black pepper to your eggs and start whisking the eggs until you get a smooth yellow consistency.

Once your minced-spice mixture looks ready, add the eggs into it and stir it. Let that simmer for two more minutes, and your breakfast or lunch is prepared.

This is a very rich dish so the combination of eggs and minced with spices are filling. But for those with a bigger appetite; they can eat this dish with the sabayad(Somali flatbread) or loxoox(Somali pancakes).

Surbiyaan – Somali Rice

Surbiyaan is an overwhelming rice dish typically eaten in Somaliland. This rice dish is prevalent on holidays such as weddings, birthdays, Islamic parties but is also made for funerals. Cooking this dish takes a bit of time, mainly because of the time needed for all the exciting ingredients of sweet, spicy, tart, and savoury to come together.

Requisites: four people
- 500g basmati rice
- 500 grams of lamb (fresh)
- 3 tomatoes
- 5 white onions

Delightful Somali recipes

- 2 red chillies
- 2/ 3 tablespoons of tomato puree
- coriander
- 4 pieces Cardamom
- 2 floury potatoes
- half tablespoon curry
- 1 bell pepper (colour does not matter)
- ½ teaspoon of green saffron
- salt
- 1 teaspoon cumin powder (cumin ground in a mortar)
- 2 cinnamon bar
- 200 grams of butter
- 3 or 4 gloves of garlic
- 1 teaspoon ground ginger (or peeled, finely chopped, and ground in mortar)
- Full cream yoghurt (3 soup spoons)
- a bit off sunflower oil

Preparation:
Cut 500 grams of organic lamb into medium-sized cubes. Do the same with two of the onions and cut the rest of the onions in natural oval shapes. Bake these oval-shaped onions in sunflower oil until they slightly turn golden brown; this process only takes a minute. If you leave the onions a bit too long in the hot oil, they might burn. Take the onions out of the oil and drain the oil out on a paper towel in a colander or a deep plate. Cover the dish off with another plate or plastic foil as you will use these onions later on. It's necessary to keep these warm.
Peel the potatoes and cut these into round, fairly thick slices; cut the tomatoes, capsicum (it does not matter which colour) in nice square cubes. Slice the red chilli peppers into fine pieces. Take two garlic gloves, peel them, and cut them into two pieces add these together with a few leaves of coriander, from which you have chopped off the stalk. You can grind the gloves together with the coriander in a mortar, or if you don't own a mortar or are not familiar with how to use it, a blender would be sufficient to get the job done.

Delightful Somali recipes

In preparation for adding the rice to the spices, wash it first and drain it before adding it to the herbs and vegetables.

Process:
Pre-head about 200 ml of sunflower oil in a stewpan, add the diced lamb meat to the pan, and stir it. Leave the meat to fry in the hot oil for approximately 3 minutes and add then the sliced onions. Bake these for a minute and a half and then add the diced tomatoes, half a teaspoon of cumin powder, sliced chilli peppers, half a teaspoon of curry powder. Mix this all together to allow the meat to soak up the different spices. After that, add two or three tablespoons of tomato puree to the mixture and leave it to fry. Finally, add the sliced potatoes and a glass of water to the meat and spices. In the meantime, boil 1 litre of water in another pan and add the Basmati rice. Add four pieces of cardamom and cinnamon sticks to the rice, the aromas released from these spices will be soaked up into the rice. Leave the rice to cook on its own without stirring because stirring will break the rice. It is also essential not to thoroughly cook the rice in the pan because it will cook further in the oven. Cooking it for about 5 minutes should be enough on low fire.
Scoop part of the sauce from the stewpan onto a bowl and cover it with a lid or plastic foil. Take cold whole cream yoghurt from the fridge and cover the remaining sauce in the stewpan with a thick layer of yoghurt without stirring it. Then scoop half of the semi-cooked rice from the pan on top of the marinated sauce in yoghurt and meat. Once again, do not stir.
Then you scoop the sauce that you had put aside on top of the rice, after this you cover this with another layer of plain yoghurt and sprinkle part of the fried onions over the yoghurt. Add the other half of the rice and finish it off by spraying a little bit of melted butter approximately 100 grams on top of the rice.
You have now basically created a sandwich consisting of two layers of sauce with the rice in between. To finish it off, add a little bit of saffron to the rice and sprinkle the remaining fried onions on top of the rice as an aesthetic gesture.

Put the lid on the pan and place the stewpan in a pre-heated oven at 180 degrees for another 20 minutes. Your meal is ready to be consumed. Because of the yoghurt component, the rice can be saved in the fridge for a maximum of two days. A day longer is technically possible, but the yoghurt goes off quickly, so it is best to enjoy it pretty quickly.

*This dish can also be made without the whole cream yoghurt.

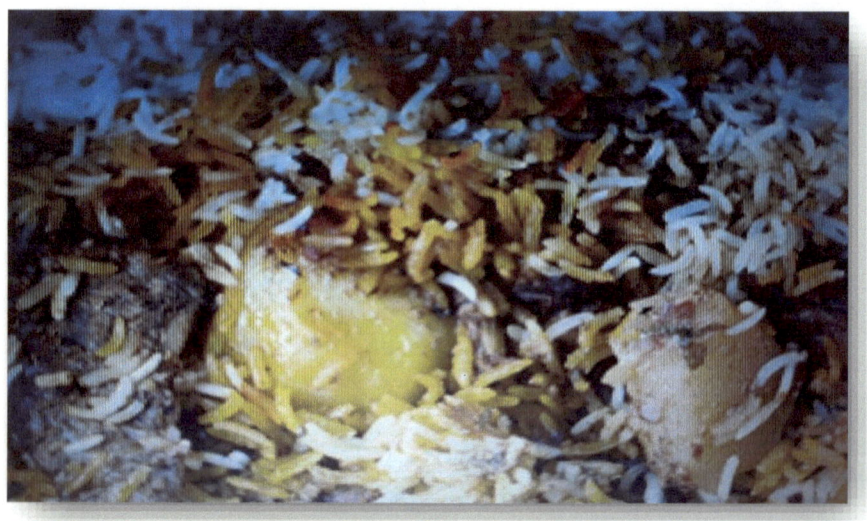

Surbiyaan rice close up

Maraq Cad – Broth with meat and vegetables

In Somaliland broth or Maraq-cad, white soup is often drawn from lamb meat with bones or camel meat. It is a spicy soup, also known as white soup, because of its colour or lack thereof. Maraq-cad also contains spices, potatoes, and other vegetables such as carrots, spring onion, onions, and white cabbage. Essentially the vegetables can be anything as long as the main

Delightful Somali recipes

ingredients are meat with bone and white cabbage, carrots, and potatoes.

Somalis then separate the broth from the meat and vegetables in a colander and serve the broth as an appetizer, like soup is an appetizer in the West. Somalis generally believe that this soup has medicinal powers due to its nutritional value. To be more precise, the general belief is that it helps your body recover faster from a common cold and reduces menstrual pain. Also, it's a popular dish amongst people who suffer from hay fever. This broth is famous amongst Somalis throughout the entire year, but it is especially popular amongst those living in the West in the winter months.

In the West, the Somalis believe that they won't catch a cold if they regularly include this broth into their diet, therefore in addition to the winter version of this dish, they often add ground ginger root. The idea is that ginger keeps your body warm in the winter, thus keeps the flue at a distance. As discussed earlier, the Maraq can be served and consumed in a variety of ways.

Necessities: 4 people
- 1 Spring onions
- 4 gloves of garlic
- 1 White cabbage
- lamb shoulder with bone or lamb leg 500 gram
- 3 large potatoes
- 2 red or white onions
- 3 green hot peppers (Thai)
- 3 carrots
- Dried coriander seeds
- 1 teaspoon of salt
- ½ teaspoon of cumin powder
- Coriander leaves

Preparation: It is vital to get a nice piece of meat with fairly enough meat on the bone for this dish. Chop the lamb shoulder

Delightful Somali recipes

or leg in large junky pieces and put that in a large soup pot. Add a bit of black pepper and salt together with garlic, onions, and tomatoes to the pool. Leave the meat to boil for 20 minutes with the lid on, as you are striving for a nice piece of soft flesh that slides of the bone.

In the meantime, wash the vegetables, peel the potatoes, spring onions and cut these in reasonably large junks. Bind the litters of cabbage with a thread to not fall apart in loose leaves while cooking. Use the green part of the spring onion for this dish and add that, together with the carrots, potatoes, and cabbage, to the broth.

Lastly, cut the green peppers finely and bake that together with ½ teaspoon of coriander seeds in a separate pan. You will need this, as you need to sprinkle these spices on top of your broth to give it a fresh crisp.

After adding the vegetables leave the broth to cook for another 20 á 30 minutes; this way, the different flavours will penetrate the flesh of the meat. As you notice, while regularly stirring, the core has become quite soft already, and to facilitate the juices getting into the meat, you can make small incisions into the flesh to boost the absorption of the flavours in the core.

Let this process cook on low fire for another 10 minutes and stir occasionally. After a while, you will notice that the water level of the broth is decreasing; this happens as the water evaporates and it is entirely normal, so just add half a cup of water to the broth and leave that to cook.

Depending on the firmness of the broth that you are after and the spiciness, you can even add a whole cup of water. If your broth becomes too watery is becomes tasteless so try to prevent that. As a final touch, sprinkle the roasted chilli and the coriander seeds on top of the broth.

You can serve the broth in a bowl, consume it like a soup, or dip pieces of the banquette in the broth for the flavour and eat it like that. Or separate the broth from the vegetables by using a colander. The vegetables and the meat can now be roasted in a pre-heated oven at 220 degrees for another 15 minutes and served independently. This dish tastes immaculate, especially if you finish it by sprinkling the roasted chilli and coriander seeds over the broth. Another way to eat this dish is with rice; either half of the broth is used for cooking the rice, or one can simply cook the rice in plain water and eat the roasted vegetables on top of that.

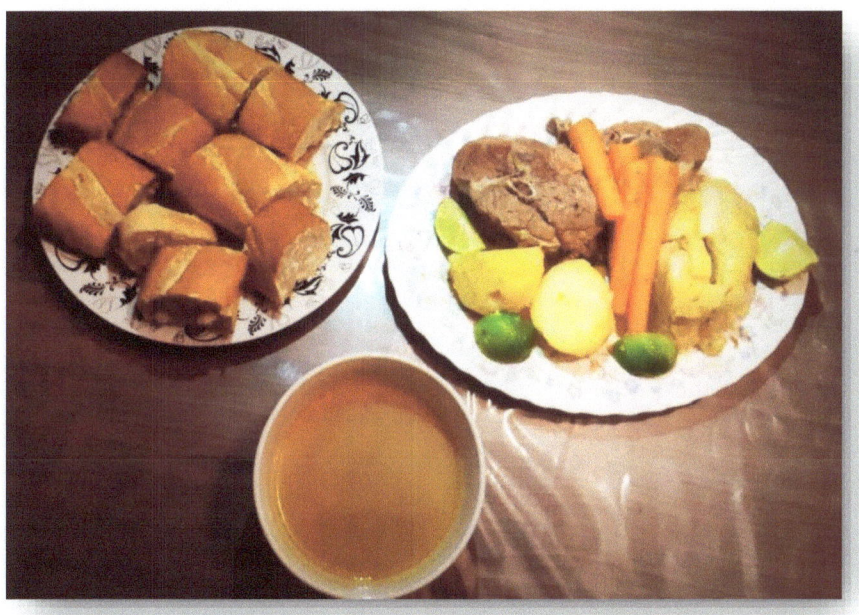

The complete Dish; Broth is separated from the meat and vegetables, and it's eaten with baguette / Sabayad

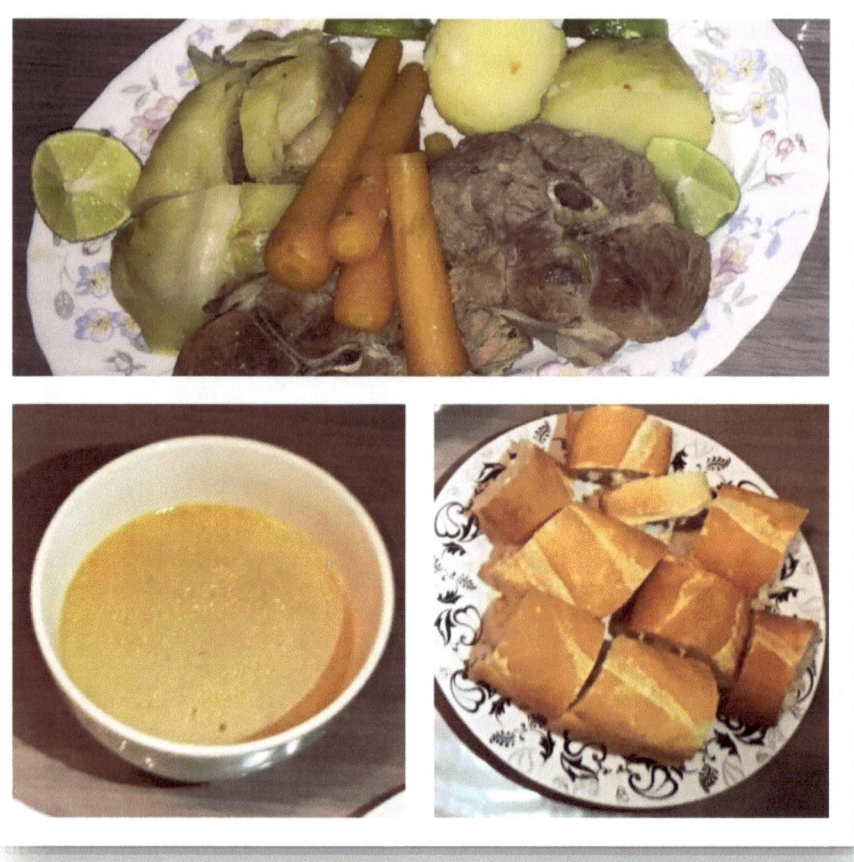

The complete Dish; Broth is separated from the meat and vegetables, and it's eaten with baguette / Sabayad

Basbaas – Hot Somali green Salsa

Basbaas is a hot Somali Salsa that is indispensable in the Somali kitchen. It is often made from hot green peppers or red peppers mixed with garlic and vinegar for preservation reasons. Vinegar is only added if Somalis are making large quantities of Basbaas and want to save it for a couple of weeks. However, it is far more common to add lemon to the peppers as it breaks the heat level yet makes the Basbaas more flavoursome.

Peppers, in general, are not just a condiment to add flavour to our food, but they also carry a few essential vitamins and minerals such as iron, magnesium, phosphorus, vitamin C, B, and E.

Cayenne pepper, in particular, also has vitamin B6, potassium, and manganese. It reduces aches and pain in the human body.

Necessities:
- 3 cayenne peppers
- 2 gloves of garlic
- 1 tablespoon of lime
- ¼ teaspoon of salt

Preparation:
Peel the garlic gloves, cut the front and back end of the cayenne peppers, then cut them in two. Place these ingredients in the spice grinder together with a tablespoon of lime and salt. Grind this mixture for a few minutes until you get a runny red paste. Place the Basbaas in glass Tupperware and keep it in the fridge.

The Basbaas is sprinkled on top of a variety of dishes, and as a consequence of that, it increases the appetite, therefore, the food intake of people. Young girls and women are often advised to refrain from overeating Basbaas to limit their consumption of food intake to prevent weight gain.

Delightful Somali recipes

Shaax – Somali tea

Somaliland is located close to the equator, and due to its hot weather, locals prefer to drink tea or coffee to beat the heat. The Somalis believe that it will make you thirstier if you drink soda or ice-cold water in tropical temperatures. Although most people are very particular about their tea, the most common way this tea is enjoyed is with sugar, milk, and spices. The following recipe is a complete version of how Somali tea is supposed to be relished.

Necessities: 4 people
- Teapot / pan
- 30 ml grams black tea
- 1 litre of water
- 8 x Cloves
- 5 x Cardamom
- 2x cinnamon stick; break the bars into smaller barks or one teaspoon cinnamon powder
- 1 teaspoon of ground ginger or peel 100gram of ginger cut it into tiny pieces (can also be crushed in a mortar to a paste)
- 100 grams of sugar or two tablespoons of brown sugar
- One cup of Whole milk, goats' milk, or camel milk

Preparation:
Fill a teapot with 4-normal cups, i.e., a large tea/coffee mug (1 litre) of water. Add the herbs to the water. Boil this on a low fire and stir it while boiling. Once the water starts boiling, it starts to bubble towards the surface; this is when you can add the milk into the mixture of black tea, spices, and water while stirring. You can do this by touch till the tea turns light brown, ½ a cup of milk should be sufficient. Half a cup should be enough to 4 cups, 250 ml of water. If there is too much milk in the tea, then the colour would be slightly off, and the tea tastes too watery, so you will know when you got the ratios right. If this has happened already, you can reverse the process by adding a little more black tea to the mixture. Leave the tea to boil for a few more minutes to give

the newly added tea the chance to draw into the mix of spices, sugar, and milk. If you like a strong cup of tea, then reduce the amount of milk to ¼ of a cup.

If you aim to make an all-inclusive tea, keep into account those that do not like sugar in their tea or are bound to dietary restrictions; you can prepare the tea without the sugar element. Moreover, if you are hosting vegans, it is better to use almond milk instead of soy milk for this tea.

Cinnamon Powder

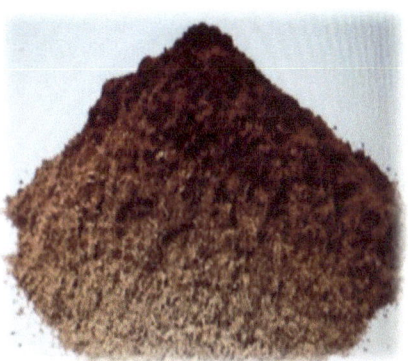

In 10 minutes, a delightful cup of tea that is also healthy can be enjoyed with friends and family.

Tip: There are various ways to prepare this tea; the above recipe is a complete version. According to personal taste, one can leave out cinnamon or ginger, or both. However, you cannot leave out the cloves and cardamom as these two ingredients are the essence of Somali tea.

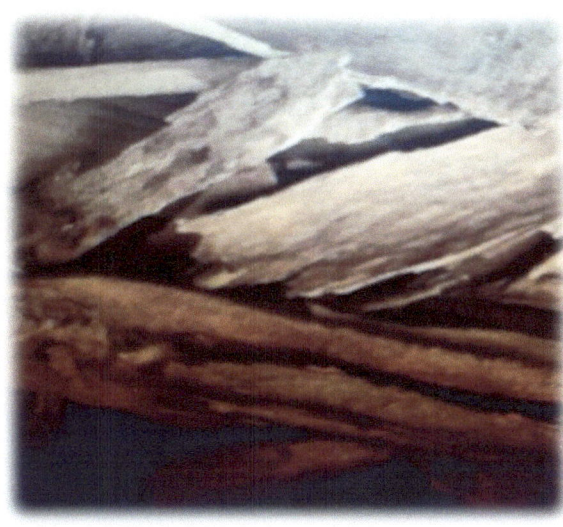

Split Cinnamon Barks

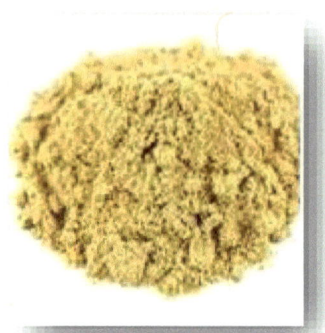

Ginger powder

Ginger Root

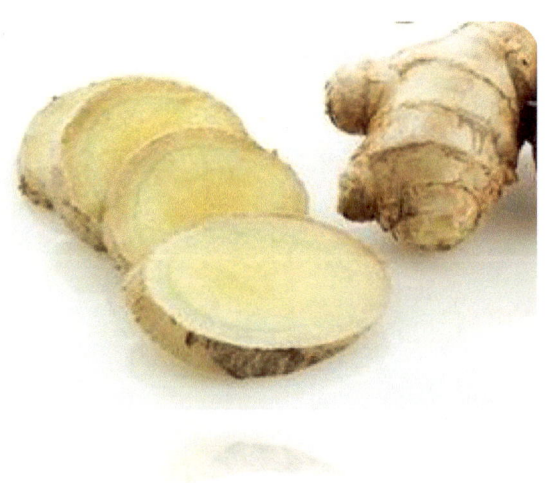

Delightful Somali recipes

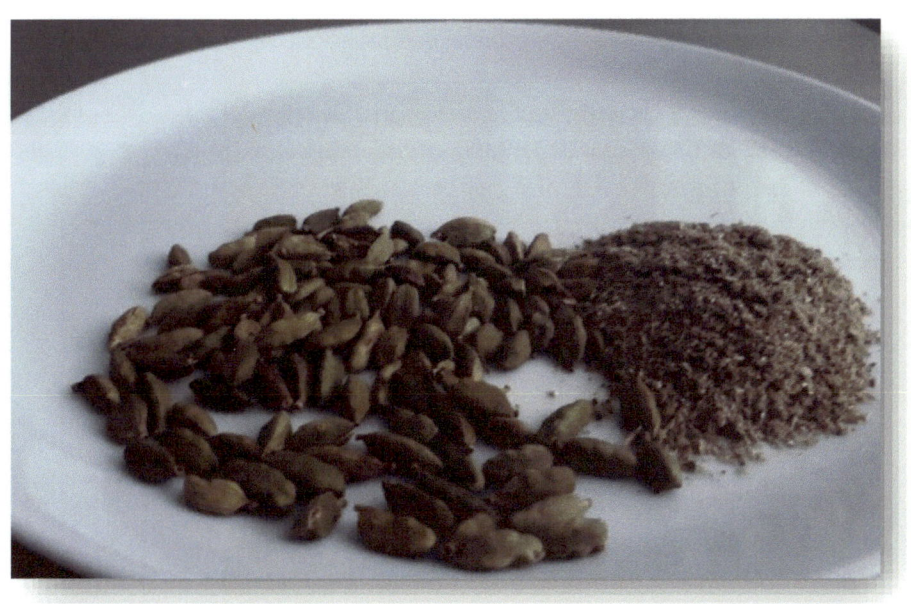

Cardamom; left whole – correct powder form

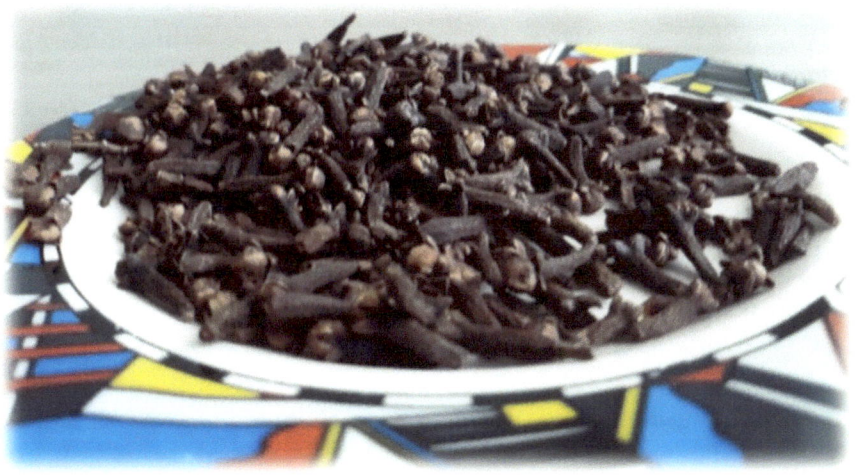

Cloves

Delightful Somali recipes

Qashar – Somali Coffee

Somaliland has a rich history of drinking instant coffee in a very unconventional way, with spices. I guess this should be the actual way of drinking coffee as the herbs contain many health benefits. Since it's a liquefied substance, your body absorbs the minerals from the spices in the coffee quicker, and therefore you will be able to enjoy the benefits earlier. Take cinnamon; it lowers your blood sugars, boosts your energy level, and stimulates brain function. It also reduces your appetite for sweet afternoon snacks, and it is an overall antidote to the cold virus as it warms up your body.

Moreover, cinnamon also harbours several beneficial minerals like magnesium, manganese, iron, fibre, several antioxidants, and vitamin K. Besides the nutritional value and increase in energy level, cinnamon also improves the taste of your coffee, just like the cardamom. Not only does cardamom add a lovely aroma to your coffee, but it also contains many health benefits, such as the reduction of high blood pressure and blood sugar. It also contains anti-inflammatory properties, and it helps against ulcers. This is excellent news for people with diabetes, mainly because cinnamon also has some of the same properties; thus, you can see this as a double-action health benefit that you can get from a single cup of coffee in the morning. However, there is more because cardamom also contains a high level of minerals such as zinc, phosphor, magnesium, potassium, and calcium. Moreover, it also has vitamins like vitamin B1, B3, B6, and vitamin C.

Necessities: 4 cups of coffee
- 250 grams Ground coffee
- 4 cups of water
- 2 cinnamon sticks (ground)
- 1 tablespoon of brown sugar
- 4 cardamom (ground)
- 5 cloves (ground)

Delightful Somali recipes

-1 cup of whole cream milk (goats milk, camel milk, almonds milk)
*small pot or a mocha pot

Preparation:
Put the spices in a food grinder and grind it until you get a powdery substance; add 250 grams of the ground coffee to the herbs and remix it. This allows the coffee and the spices to mix well. Boil this magical substance together with 4 cups of water in a pot. Adding sugar is optional, but a tablespoon of brown sugar gives the coffee a subtle sweet taste, especially when added while the mixture of coffee and spices are boiling together. Once the water starts bubbling up to the surface, add ½ a cup of whole cream milk or soy or another type of milk to it. Leave it to boil for two more minutes on shallow water.
If you use the mocha pot to make this coffee, scoop the coffee and spice mix out of the food processor, place it in the funnel, and fill the water till the edge of the valve. Put sugar or milk later on according to your preference. For a vegan diet, almond milk is preferred.

If you do not want any milk or sugar in your coffee, you can simply leave those elements out, and your coffee will still contain all the goodness you need to start your day.

Delightful Somali recipes

Buskud – Somali Tea biscuits

Somali biscuits are often made for and consumed on special occasions where the community comes together, such as Muslim festivities and Eid parties. They are also very popular on birthdays, baby showers, bachelorettes, and weddings; as long as there is a Somali crowd, these biscuits will do very well.
Suppose there is a community get-together or an occasion where there is some sort of Muslim celebration. In that case, the Somali organisers often build the anticipation up by announcing that Somali food and sweet delicacies will be served at that party. That is usually the only way, especially in foreign places where displaced Somalis live, to lure as many Somalis as possible to your party.

In this book, I am going to share the most straightforward Somali biscuit recipe. These biscuits are light, not very sweet, and delicious, especially in combination with the Xalwad. You take two biscuits and place the Xalwad in between and eat it as a sandwich. Somali children often eat these biscuits in that way.

Necessities:
- 250 grams of plain flour
- 1 teaspoon of baking powder
- 250 grams of melted butter or Somali butter
- ½ teaspoon of salt
- 1 teaspoon of vanilla extract
- 2 egg
- 150 grams of sugar grinded

Preparation:
Mix the butter with the sugar in a food processor. Once the structure starts changing and you get a paste-like substance, add the eggs and continue mixing with the food processor. Let the mixing continue for approximately five more minutes, then add

the flour, one teaspoon of baking powder, half a teaspoon of salt, one teaspoon of vanilla extract, one teaspoon of lime juice. In the meantime, grind 150 grams of white sugar until the structure changes into a powdery substance. Add the sugar powder to the mixture in the food processor and mix it for another 5 minutes. Once the mixture is done, place the dough in a cookie press and choose a front shape that you would want the cookies to take. Press the cookie dough on a pre-oiled oven plate and place the biscuits in a pre-heated oven for 20 minutes at 180 degrees. Let these biscuits cool off for approximately ten more minutes. These buttery yet dry biscuits are delicious as an afternoon snack.

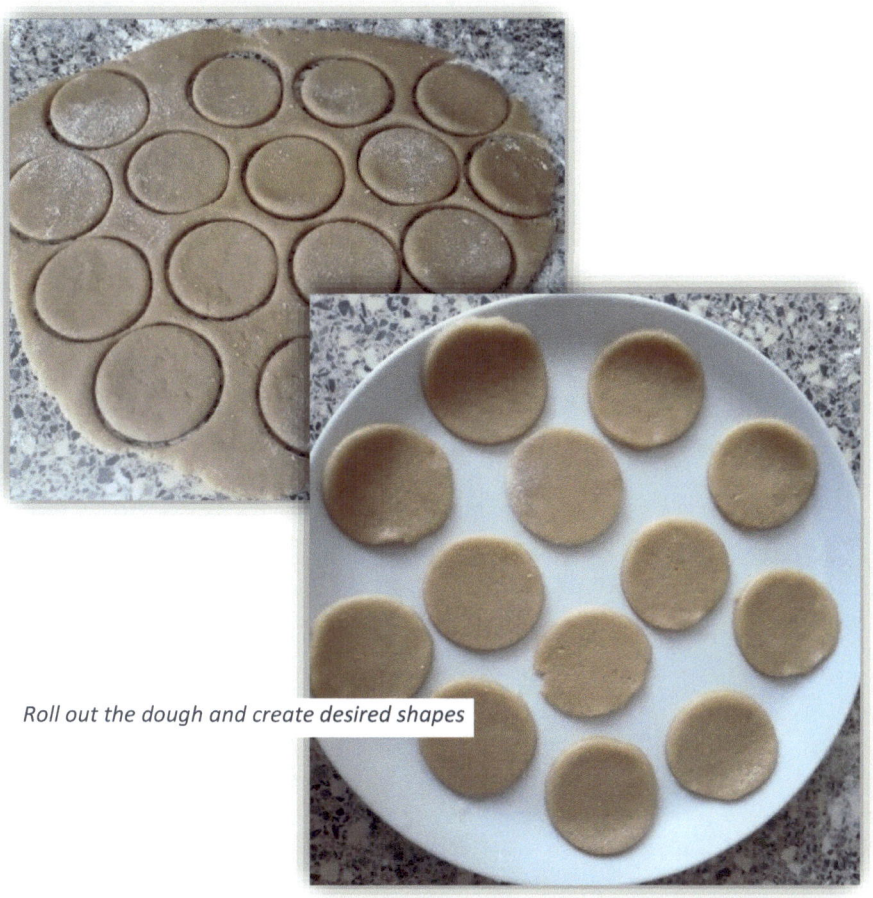

Roll out the dough and create desired shapes

Delightful Somali recipes

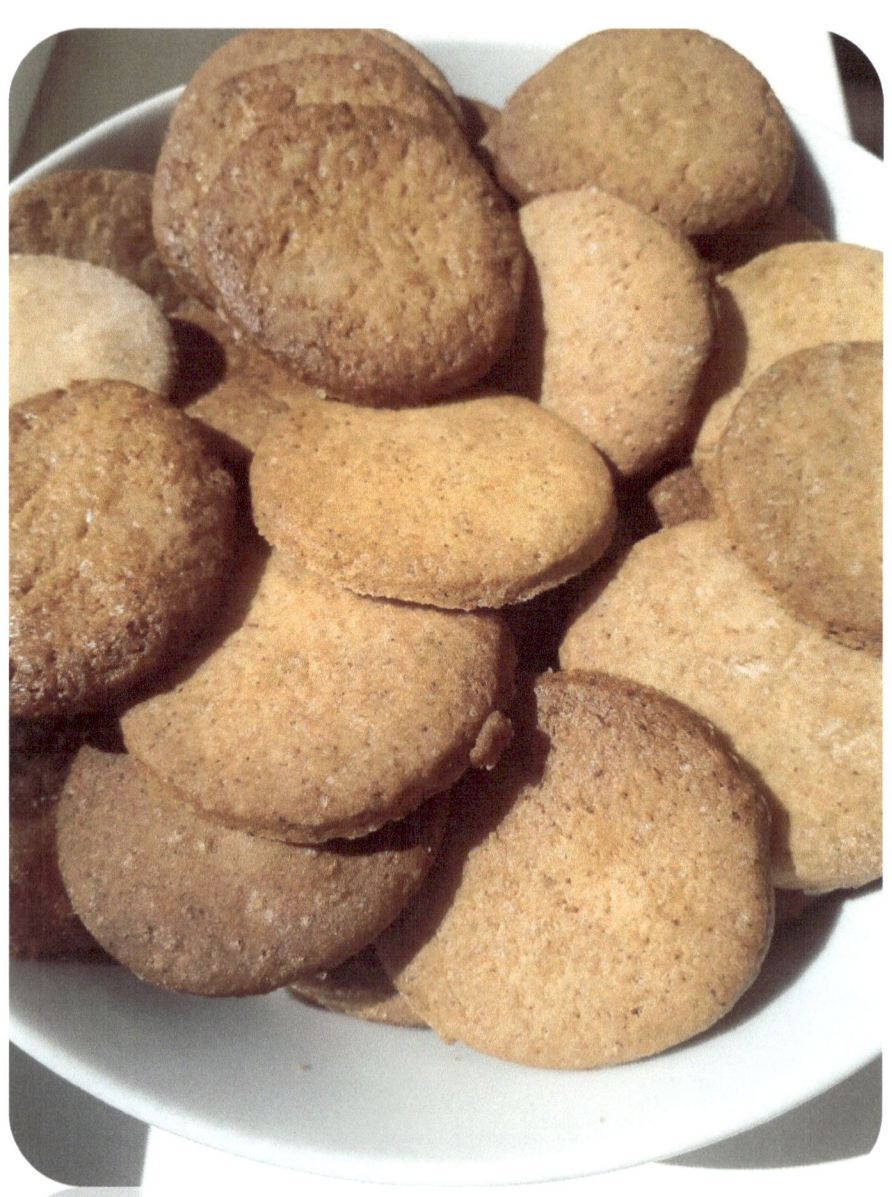

Baked Somali Tea-Bicuits (Buskud Shaax)

Delightful Somali recipes

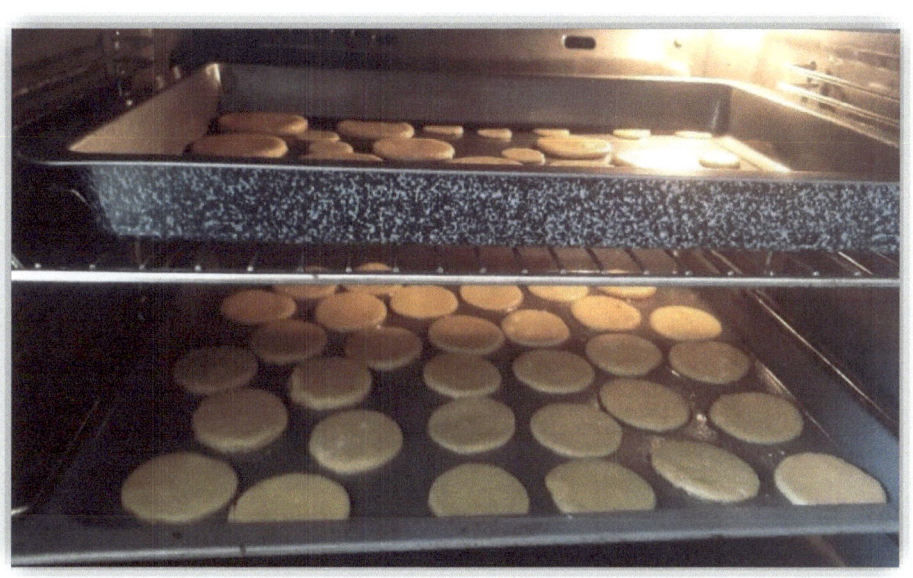

Bake for 20 to 25minutes in pre-heated oven

Delightful Somali recipes

Xalwad – Sweet dessert

The letter H in the Somali language is written as an X because there is no H in the Somali alphabet. Xalwad is a Somali delicacy often eaten on birthdays, weddings, and other celebrations. The structure looks like a brownish gel substance similar to jello on the outside, but the Xalwad is thicker.

Necessities:
- Nutmeg 3 or 4 (grounded)
- 150 grams ground cardamom
- unsalted butter or Somali butter
- canola oil/ sunflower oil
- White sugar 1.5 kg
- Black tea (1 cup)
- corn starch 250 kg
- 2 litter water
- Saffron 1 thee spoon of food colour
- red food colour ½ teaspoon
*Deep pan
*wooden spatula to stir with, preferably a long one, so you do not get burned

Preparation:
Boil 2 litres of water in a pan and 1.5 kg of white sugar and bring it to a boil. While this boiling is happening, put 250 grams of corn-starch in a bowl together with a teaspoon of saffron and the red food colouring in the bowl and one cup of pre-cooked strong black tea (250 ml).
Mix this well by hand using a whisk or with an electronic mixer. Either way, make sure there are no lumps in the corn-starch mix. Add the bright coloured corn-starch mix to the mixture of boiling water and sugar and stir it well to avoid any lumps once again. After about 10 minutes, you will see the consistency change as it becomes thicker; add 100 grams of sunflower or canola oil to

prevent the corn starch from sticking to the bottom of the sides of the pan. After approximately 15 minutes, you need to add another 100 ml of oil while stirring. Now you can leave it to boil on medium heat and stir every 5 minutes or so. Make sure you put a lid on the pan because when the mixture of corn-starch, sugar, and oil starts boiling its starts bubbling up, and it may come onto your skin, which in essence can burn your skin.
As the consistency becomes firmer and thicker, you will notice large bubbles come about; you will need to add about 100 grams of butter to the texture to smoothen it out.

After a while, you will notice that it's becoming more difficult to stir the mixture as the mixture changes into a thick brownish coherent substance. Add 100 grams of butter to the now percolating sense to soften the structure. After another 30 minutes, add another 100 grams of butter to the mixture for an even smoother texture and a pleasant smell.

In the meantime, place approximately 4 or 5 pieces of cardamom in a blender and grind it. Remove the shell from the nutmegs and crush it until a fine powdery substance comes about. Add this gel-like mixture and stir it profusely; this will allow the butter and the corn starch to soak up the spices. Keep stirring it every 5 minutes.

After another 20 minutes, you will see that the butter has melted nicely into the mixture but that the oil has been separated onto the surface of the Xalwad. Separate this excess oil from the Xalwad by scooping it out of the pan. Or use a sieve to remove the extra fat from the oil but make sure you boil under the sieve to preserve the Xalwad if it falls out of the colander/sieve.

After removing the extra oil from the Xalwad, you need to remove it from the stove and leave it to cool for about an hour.

Before taking it off the heat and after the excess oil has been removed, you can choose to sprinkle roasted peanuts on top of

Delightful Somali recipes

the Xalwad and stir it to mix the peanuts evenly throughout the Xalwad mix. The roasted peanuts are optional as the Xalwad is lovely on its own. Yet another aesthetically pleasing way to serve this dessert is to leave out the roasted peanuts and sprinkle some sesame seeds on top of the Xalwad after being cooled.

The latter does not change the taste of the Xalwad; it just looks better when presented.

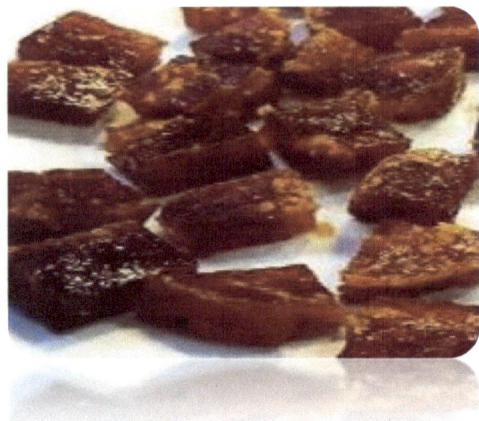
Xalwad

Delightful Somali recipes

Sambusa – Savoury Treat

Somali Sambusa is a hearty triangle snack often eaten during the iftar meal to break the fast after a day of fasting in the month of Ramadan. The outside is made from a thin layer of dough, while the inside consists of hot green chilli pepper, white onion cubes, and mince. However, Sambusa has turned into the favourite

street food for many people in the West as it can easily be turned into an entire meal by increasing its size. The normal Sambusa is as big as half of a small envelope, contrary to the large ones who are as big as the whole small envelope

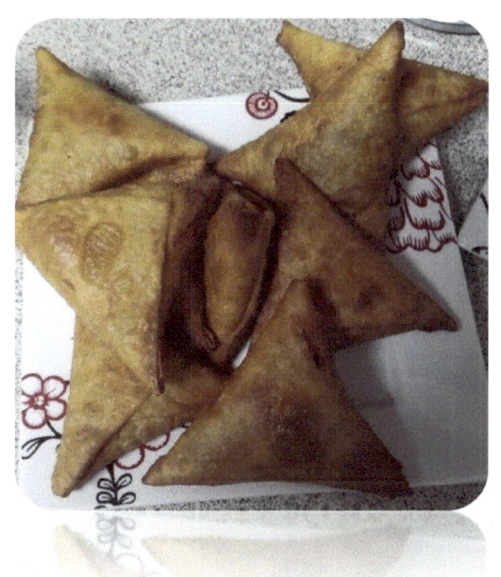

Amenities: the content of the Sambusa
- 5 large white onions
- 250 grams of minced ground beef
- 200 grams of butter / 50 ml vegetable oil
- 3 green bell peppers
- 4 gloves of garlic
- 2 serrano's / cayenne peppers
- 3 stalks of coriander
- 2 teaspoons of cumin powder
- 1 teaspoon of salt
* pan

Pastry:
- 250-gram plain flower
- 150 ml water
- 100 ml of vegetable / canola oil

Prepare the content of the Sambusa.
Dry boil the mincemeat in a saucepan until it releases all its
moisture. Add butter to the mince and ground garlic or a mix of
garlic and coriander paste mixed in the mortar. Bake it for about
5 minutes, add cumin powder, salt, and finely chopped cayenne
or serrano peppers to the mixture and bake it while adding about
50 ml of vegetable oil into the mix. Slice the bell peppers into
small cubes and add these to the mincemeat mix; lastly, chop the
coriander leaves refined and add these to the saucepan. Leave
this mixture of mince and spices to cook until there is no more
moisture left in there. Separate the excess oil from the saucepan
by dipping a large spoon in the pan and taking out the extra fat.
You aim for a grease-free mince, vegetables, and spice mixture
that you can use as content for your Sambusa, the triangle-
shaped pastry.

Pastry:
The pastry part of the Sambusa is made the same way as the
Somali flatbread – Sabayad but thinned out more by rolling it out
even more. Then you divide the square into four pieces and fold it
into triangles.

Another more practical option and very common in the West is to
buy square-shaped filo dough and cut that into four pieces. Filo
dough is a fragile dough that tears easily, and especially when it's
going to be fried in pre-heated oil, this dough might absorb too
much fat, and your Sambusa might get entrenched(infused) with
oil. A greasy Sambusa is what you are trying to prevent. So, in this
case, it is better to layer two or even three filo dough sheets and
cut the square up into four pieces, and use that for one Sambusa.

Take a small bowl and place a little bit of plain flour in there; add
a minimum amount of water, for example, a tablespoon, and mix

Delightful Somali recipes

it well. This substance is sticky, and you can use it to attach the ends of the squares when folding into a triangle.

Step 1

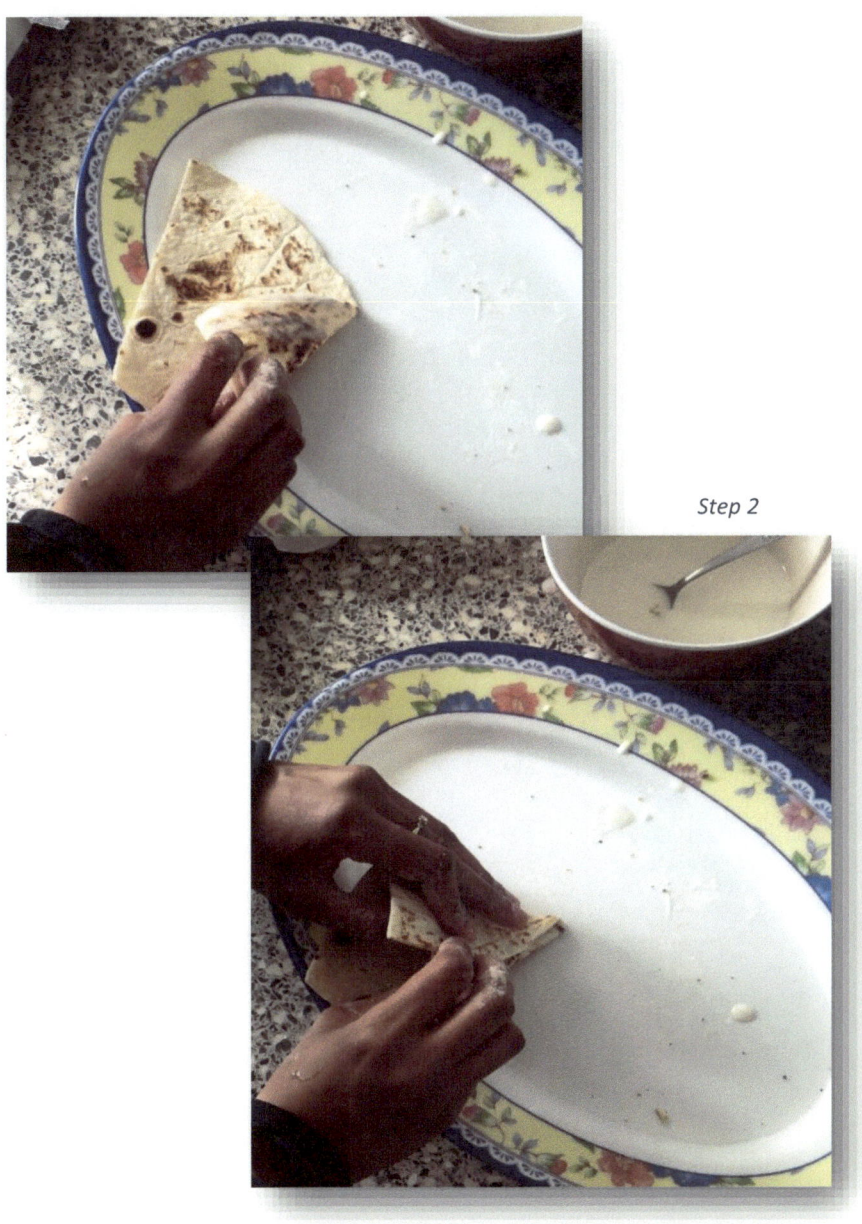

Step 2

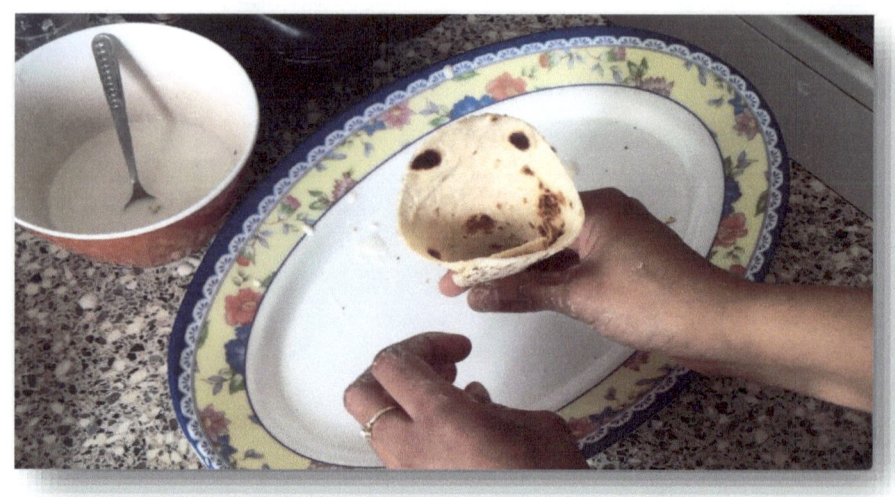

Step 3: Upside down triangle shape

Step 4: Fill the Sambusa with the minced & spices

Step 5: Close the Sambusa off by creasing the **inside and folding the outher triangle**

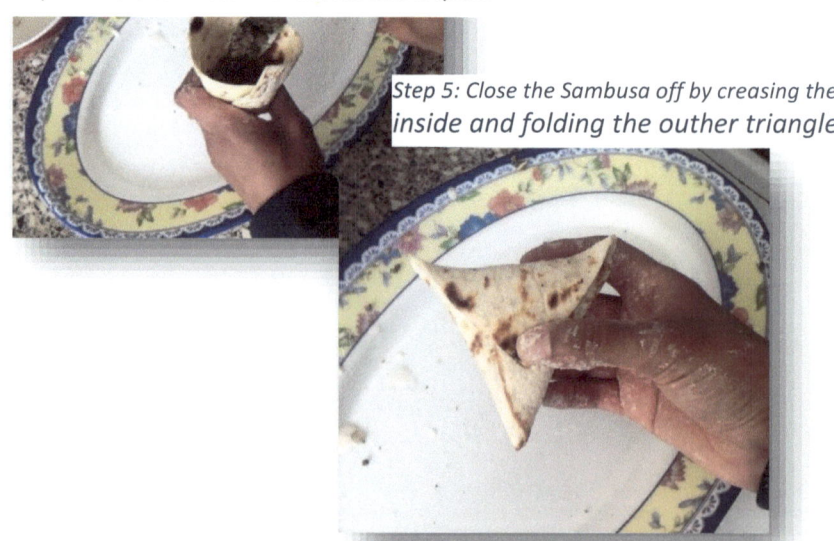

Delightful Somali recipes

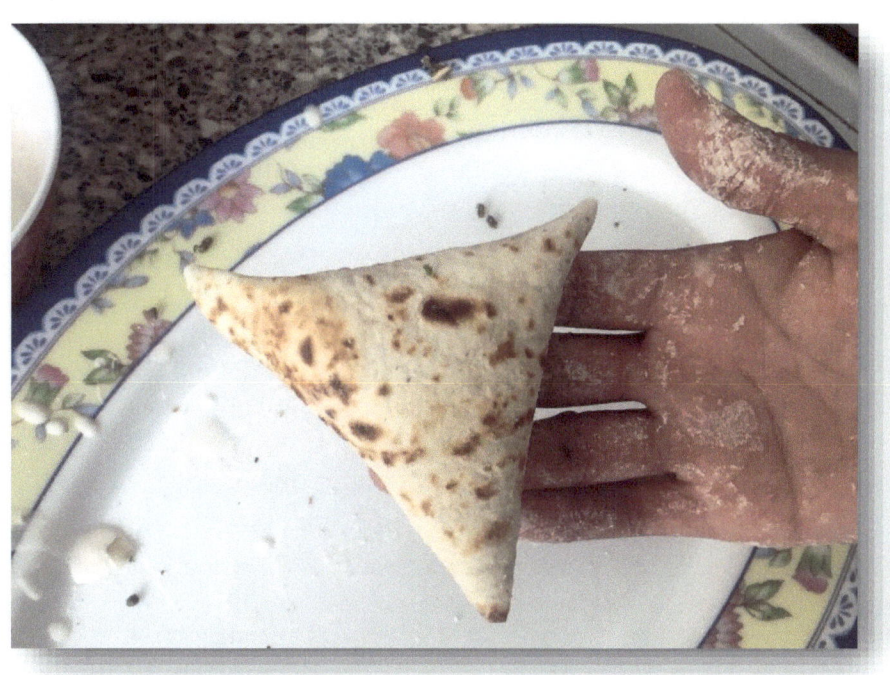

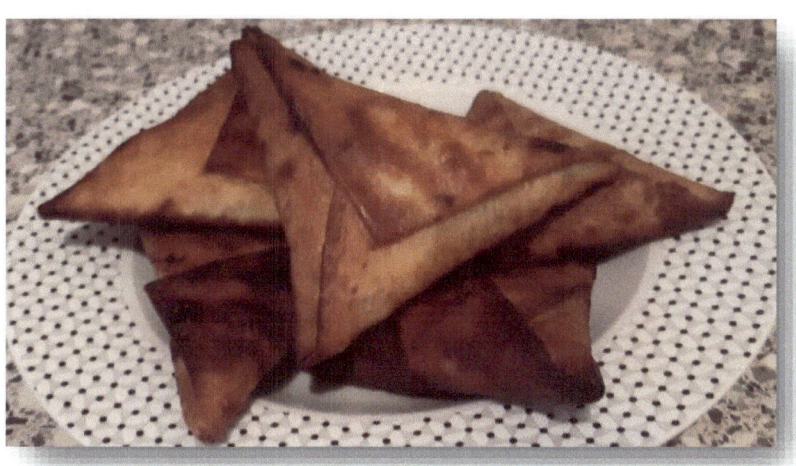

Final result; Fried Sambusa

Delightful Somali recipes

Muqmad – Preserved "Jerky" Camel Meat

Muqmad is jerky meat made from camel meat eaten with Somali pancakes for breakfast or dinner and dates at weddings. It is not common to eat this dish as a regular meal because it takes a lot of time and energy to prepare it. The Muqmad is made from small cubicles of dried camel meat. Essentially Muqmad is eaten at national festivals or weddings with a paste made from dates and butter. This dish is trendy amongst Somali men.
For this dish, it's essential to use lean meat with the least amount of fat on it, for example, the meat cut from the leg of the camel. The core must be non-fat lean meat; otherwise, you cannot make Muqmad out of it. To enjoy this dish longer, one needs to preserve it in a vacuum jar together with a bit of a mix of spiced butter and oil.

In the original recipe, the idea is to cut the meat into small cubicles, dry it in the sun for half a day and then fry it in butter or sunflower oil. However, it is hard to get camel meat in the West, so lean beef meat from a grass-fed animal will do. Moreover, instantly cooking the meat instead of first drying it in natural sunlight is more suitable for western standards.

*This recipe is the western version.

Amenities: 6 people
- 2 kg of lean Beef meat or Camel meat
- Sunflower oil 250 ml
- Butter or Somali butter
- Ground cardamom (100 ml)
- Ground black pepper (1 teaspoon)
- Salt

Date paste:
- 2 kg of dates
- ½ teaspoon of ground black pepper

- 1 teaspoon of ground cardamom
* stew pot
* frying pan
* large bowl

Preparations:
Cook the meat cubicles in a stew pot in a little bit of water, add a teaspoon of salt, ½ teaspoon of ground black pepper. Leave it to cook in the pan for approximately 10 minutes until the meat releases all the blood and moisture. When that has happened, drain the aliment with a strainer, make sure all the moist is gone from the meat before you start frying it in sunflower oil in a pre-heated pot on medium heat.

Fry the meat together with a teaspoon of ground cardamom for 10 minutes on medium heat until it changes colour from grey to dark brown. Once again, strain the oil out of the meat, leave the meat to dry, and cool off on a paper towel. The paper towel will soak up the excess grease out of the flesh.

Melt about 300 grams of butter in another pan on medium heat and add about ½ teaspoon cardamom to the oil. Let this bake for about 5 to 7 minutes, and add 100ml of sunflower oil to the mixture. Let this mixture bake until the mixture starts turning into a light brown coherent fluid mix.

Take a bowl and place the meat cubes together with the brownish mixture of butter and oil.

Now we can start the second part of the dish. Cut about 2 kilograms of dates in halves and remove the pits; throw out the dates that are too dry or have gone wrong.

Place the dates in a bowl and mould them with your hands into a paste. Add a spoon of the brownish oil mixture together with ½ teaspoon of ground black pepper and a ½ teaspoon of ground cardamom. Knead the dates and spices until a thick, supple paste comes about.

Delightful Somali recipes

Dates

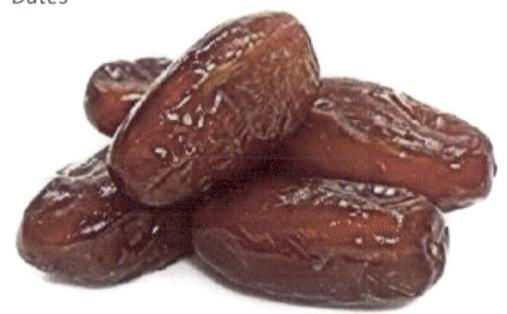

Cut the paste off with your hands and roll it in the palm of your hands making circular motions into small or medium-sized rounds squashed together dates come to existence.

Muqmad - Dry Camel Meat

Scoop the beef pieces on a plate and do the same with the ball-shaped dates pieces.
You can now eat the dates together with the jerky meat. The Muqmad can also be enjoyed on a pancake, loxoox together with black tea, or on a Sabayad.

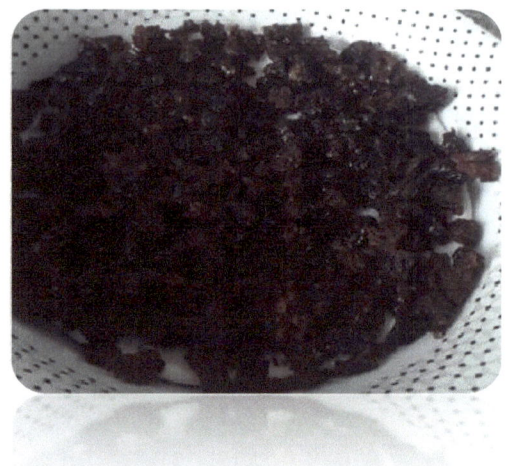

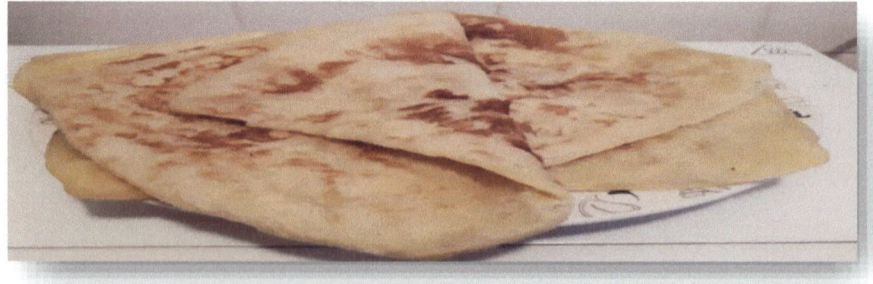

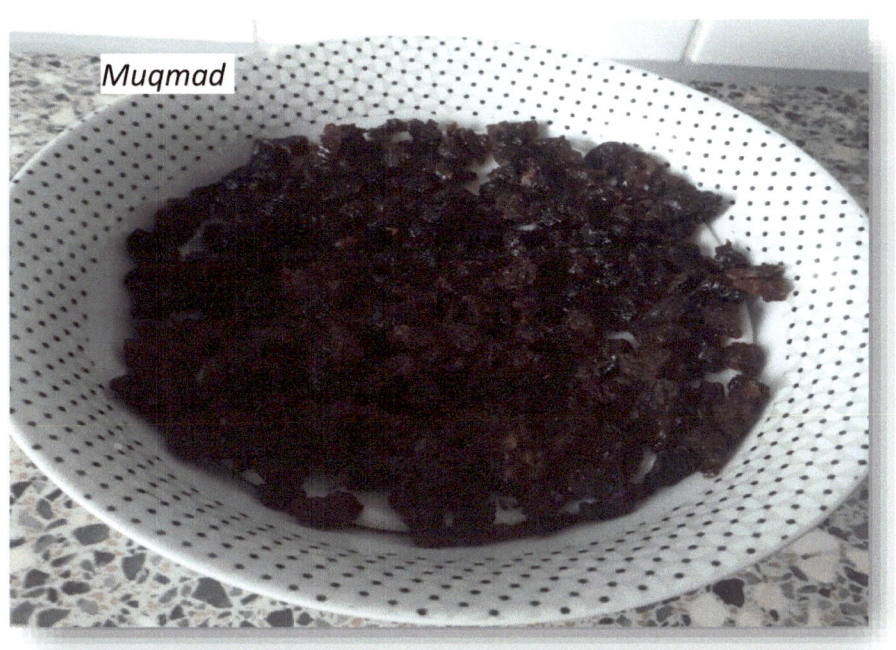

Muqmad

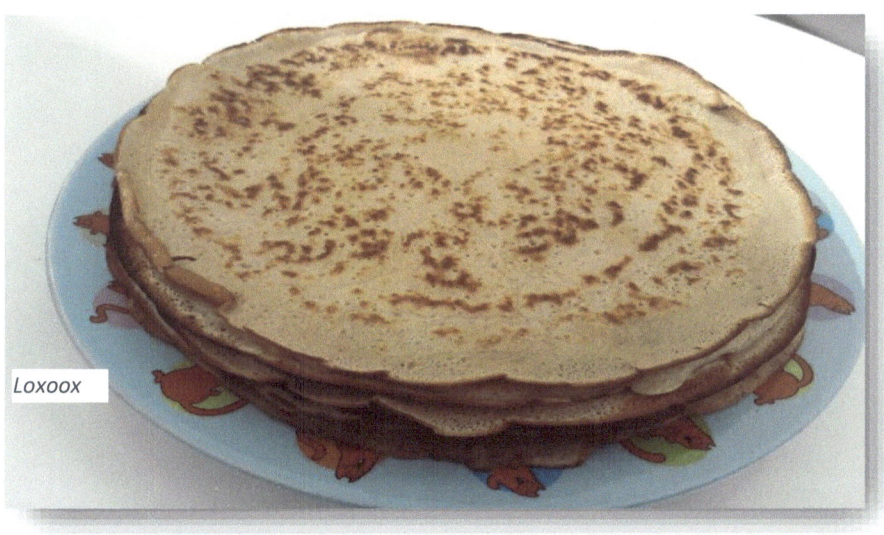

Loxoox

Delightful Somali recipes